Remembering God *and* Reminding Others

Jean Melson

WESTBOW
PRESS®
A DIVISION OF THOMAS NELSON
& ZONDERVAN

This book is a work of non-fiction. Unless otherwise noted, the author and the publisher make no explicit guarantees as to the accuracy of the information contained in this book and in some cases, names of people and places have been altered to protect their privacy.

WestBow Press books may be ordered through booksellers or by contacting:

WestBow Press
A Division of Thomas Nelson & Zondervan
1663 Liberty Drive
Bloomington, IN 47403
www.westbowpress.com
844-714-3454

Scripture taken from the New King James Version®. Copyright © 1982 by Thomas Nelson. Used by permission. All rights reserved.

ISBN: 978-1-6642-0655-7 (sc)
ISBN: 978-1-6642 0799-8 (e)

Print information available on the last page.

WestBow Press rev. date: 09/30/2020

FOREWORD

This book started as letters to an unknown friend. I was told she needed encouragement. Her life was filled with so much unhappiness she would sometimes just forget the joy and peace that was available to her. So, I wrote letters to her, to remind her of God's power, love and peace. Now these letters have been turned into a book to help you remember. Stroll with me down memory lane, walk with me through God's creation and open His word with me and let's explore ways in which we can remember God.

I would like to dedicate this book to my sister, Linda Kay Kingsley. Thanks for always being there.

I love you!

CONTENTS

Getting Started xiii

Chapter 1   Butterflies 1
Chapter 2   Wind 6
Chapter 3   Lights 10
Chapter 4   Sticks and Twigs 15
Chapter 5   Singing 20
Chapter 6   Birds 25
Chapter 7   Mirrors 30
Chapter 8   Rainbows 34
Chapter 9   Rocks 40
Chapter 10   Bookmarks 45
Chapter 11   Flowers and Herbs 49
Chapter 12   Rods and Needles 54
Chapter 13   Water 59

A Last Few Words 63
Biography 65

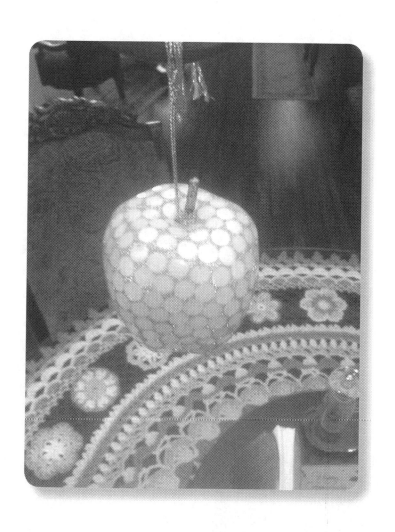

GETTING STARTED

APPLES OF GOLD

It was the style back during the time of the civil war and on into the nineteen thirties and forties for young women to wear lockets with a picture or lock of hair of their sweetheart in them. My mother had such a locket and my dad put her picture in it and took it with him when he went oversees in WW ll. Now I have her locket and when I wear it, I remember her and my dad and the love they had for each other.

When I hold her Bible in my hands, I remember her. When we set the table with her dishes, I remember her. When I was just a kid, she gave me a golden apple Christmas ornament. It came with a scripture attached, ***A word fitly spoken is like apples of gold in settings of silver.*** (Proverbs 25:11) She gave it to me to remind me to watch my mouth! Today, it hangs from the chandelier over our dinning table. When I look at it, I remember her and the admonition of King Solomon.

When I look at her photographs, when we sing her favorite hymns in worship services, I remember my mom.

Women are busy creatures. Our day to day lives are full of activity from the time we get up until we go to bed. Husbands, children, and for some, grandchildren or parents, jobs, school, housework, laundry. And then there are after school activities, and hobbies, not only our own, but everyone elses too. And the list goes on and on. Occasionally, we do something just to fill time, like watch a stupid television show we don't even like!

Is there a way in all of this activity to remember God? We have lockets, photographs, dishes and other mementos to remind us of loved ones. What reminds us of God? Do we look for those reminders, hold them close to help us remember?

One Sunday after services, I conducted a survey. I asked men and women both, what reminded them of our Heavenly Father. Some of the answers I expected, some surprised me. Here are some of the answers.

The most common answer was nature. Another one I heard as lot; a new baby. Some others were:

A storm	The view out my window
My church family	The sea shore
Baby kittens	My Bible
My morning walk	A garden
The sunset	A gentle rain
The fact that I exist	My horses and dogs
The mountains	Natures cycle of life
A snow fall	The 23 Psalm

One lady said she couldn't explain why, but whenever she smelled a cake or cookies baking, she always thought of God.

Two hundred and sixty seven times in scripture, the word remember or remembrance appears. It must be important. A lot of these verses tell us God remembers us. We are told He watches over us, cares for us, provides for us and hears our prayers. Other verses tell us to remember Him. Remember all He has done and continues to do.

Solomon told us to remember God, not once a year, not even once a week on Sunday, but every day, all day, as long as we live! ***Remember your Creator in the days of your youth.*** He continued on to tell us to remember God during the hard times that come into every life and to remember God as we grow into our later years. Then he said ***Remember your Creator before the silver card is loosed*** (the end of your life, it will be too late then). ***Then their dust will return to the earth as it was, And the spirit will return to God who gave it.*** (Ecclesiastes 12:1-7)

God has provided all His wondrous creation to remind us that He is the One True Jehovah God. But He has also provided something else. His words, written down and preserved for us. It began with Moses, when he wrote the words of the Lord. (Exodus 24: 4)

The Lord spoke to Jeremiah and told him to write down ***"all the words***

I spoke to you, from the days of Josiah even to this day" (Jeremiah 36:2) Moses and Jeremiah wrote down God's history book for us.

Later, Luke said he wrote an orderly account of the life of Christ. (Luke1:3)

John wrote, he was *the disciple who testifies of these things, and wrote of all these things concerning Jesus.* (John 21:24)

The apostle Paul wrote to the church in Rome: *whatever things were written before were written for our learning.* (Romans 15:4)

The apostle Peter wrote, *I will be careful to ensure that you always have a reminder of these things.* (2 Peter 1:15) What things? All the things he had witnessed in the life of Christ. All that He said and did. And because of the Holy Spirit, we do have the writings of scripture, things written by Moses, the prophets, the apostles and all the other writers, preserved for us and for all future generations.

These are the words of the Lord: *"Hear oh Israel: the Lord our God, the Lord is one! You shall love your God with all your heart, with all your soul and with all your might! And these words which I command you today shall be in your heart; you shall teach them diligently to your children, and you shall talk of them when you sit in your house, when you walk by the way, when you lie down, and when you rise up. You shall bind them as a sign on your hand* (bracelets) *and they shall be as frontlets between your eyes* (headbands). *You shall write them on your door posts of your house and on your gates."* (Deuteronomy 6:4-9)

Not only does the Lord tell us to remember, but He commands us to remind others! Diligently teach our children, every day! Teach others as we walk through each day. The words of the Lord should be on our minds first thing in the morning and the last thing at night.

We have Bibles in every room. We tape scripture to mirrors, we hang pictures and plaques with scripture printed on them. Some of us wear jewelry with scripture inscribed. Some of us have golden apples hanging over our tables. Do we take time to look at them? To read them? Or are we so busy we just walk past them?

What reminds you of God? Do you remind others?

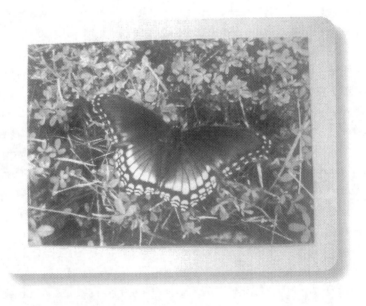

One

BUTTERFLIES

"Happiness is a butterfly, which when pursued, is always just beyond your grasp, but which if you will sit down quietly, may alight upon you."

Nathaniel Hawthorn

Did you know there are more then twenty eight thousand species of butterflies? The mystery and beauty of these creatures have always stirred the emotions of humans. Every culture has traditions, myths and beliefs concerning butterflies.

On the first of November, the people of Mexico celebrate "Dia de los Muetos", the day of the dead. This is the time of migration for the Monarch butterflies. They return to Mexico for the winter and the people believe these monarchs are the souls of their dead ancestors returning for the celebration.

In Greek mythology also, butterflies were believed to be the souls of the dead. Chinese tradition says the butterfly represents eternal life or immortality. The Japanese people believe butterflies are the symbol of love and happiness. Still others believe butterflies to be the symbol of change or new life.

American Indians have their own traditions that change from tribe to tribe. For some, butterflies bring dreams. For others, they bring joy. Some believe the butterfly is symbolic of young girl changing into a woman. For some, butterflies bring hope.

If you search your Bible, you will find no mention of butterflies. None!

But the Bible does have a lot to say about many of the teachings found in these myths and traditions.

There are scriptures concerning the newness and shortness of life. James, the brother of Christ, asked this question, ***What is your life? Is is as a vapor that appears for a little while and then vanishes away.*** (James 4:14) There are scriptures that speak of death. ***And it is appointed for men to die once, but after this the judgment.*** (Hebrews 9:27) And some speak of our immortality. When Paul wrote to Timothy, he told him: When Jesus came, ***He abolished death and brought life and immortality to light through the gospel.*** (2 Timothy 1:10) When Paul wrote to Titus he said ***we have hope of eternal life which God, who cannot lie, promised before time began.*** (Titus 1:2)

Other scriptures tells us of joy, peace, happiness and transformation.

Transformation: Metamorphosis, change, becoming different -

As the butterfly goes through metamorphosis, it's change is visible. We can watch it become a thing of beauty. So also, we can change; becoming women of Godly beauty.

King David prayed, ***"Create in me new heart, Oh, God and renew a steadfast (faithful) spirit in me."***(Psalm 51:10)

The apostle Paul said **"If any one is in Christ, he is a new creature; old things are passed away; behold, all things have become new'** (2 Corinthians 5:17) He wrote to the church in Rome, ***Do not be conformed to this world, but be transformed by the renewing of your mind***. (Romans 12:2) He tells us, once we become a Christian we have a new, clean beginning and our transformation is the result of a new way of thinking.

King David asked for a clean, new, different heart. Paul tells us to renew our minds, start over, be new in our thinking. It is all a matter of heart and mind. As my dad would say. "It's all about attitude." You have to want to be different, because it will be quite a change.

Change is visible. If you loose weight, dye your hair or get new clothes, everyone notices the difference. And if you become a new woman in Christ, your change is visible! You are being transformed, the Spirit of God is dwelling in you and you look different. Others look at you and see love and joy in you. They see peace in you. They see patience and kindness in you. They see goodness in you. They see faithfulness and gentleness, and they see self-control in you. (Galatians 5:22-23) What do these things look like?

LOVE - to love someone means you want only what is best for that person
  love your enemies, Matthew 5:44-46
  love your neighbor, Matthew 19:19
  love your husbands and your children, Titus 2:4
  love not only in words, but in deeds, 1 John 3:18
JOY - gladness of heart, absence of the weight of guilt
  being joyful when you resist or overcome temptation, James 1:2-3
  be joyful even in times of trial and poverty 2 Corinthians 8:2
PEACE - absence of conflict, contentment, mutual harmony
  your peace comes from God Philippians 4:7
  strive for peace with everyone, Romans 12:18
LONGSUFFERING - patient, the ability to suppress annoyance
  teaching with patience, 2 Timothy 4:2
  be patient with those who are indebted to you, Matthew 18:23-35
KINDNESS - benevolence, charity, sympathy, compassion
  being kind, even to those who don't receive it or thank you for it,
  Luke 6:35
GOODNESS - moral excellence, virtue, honesty, accomplishing good
  to be full of goodness, Galatians 6:10
FAITHFULNESS - being true to your vow, determined, loyal, devoted,
  steadfast
  faithfully do....continue to do good, 3 John 5
  never stop doing the work of the Lord, 1 Corinthians 15:58
  steadfast in the faith, 1 Peter 5:9
GENTLENESS - feelings of tenderness, non-abrasive
  the opposite of quarreling, 2 Timothy 2:24
  gentle toward everyone, Titus 3:2
SELF CONTROL - to be in control of one's actions or thoughts
  control your tongue, James 1:26
  control your thoughts, Hebrews 4:12
  control your body, 1 Corinthians 9:27
  put away all anger, Ephesians 4:31

Don't let me mislead you here. This transformation is not "a one time, over night, now I've done it, what's next?" thing. We are to have a change of heart. But, just as a butterfly struggles to become a thing of beauty, so we will struggle to change. It isn't easy! Old habits die hard. Paul wrote to the church in Corinth ***The inward man is being renewed day by day.*** (2 Corinthians 4:16) Day by day, not over night. Don't give up! When you begin to change the way you think about things, your attitude will begin to change. Your actions will begin to change. What is right, what is wrong? What is important, what isn't? What is true, what isn't?

This will be a long metamorphosis. The butterfly shows change every minute of every day, she works hard at it, until her metamorphosis is complete. We should show change every minute of every day. It is hard, but with God's help it can be done! We should grow more like Him every day until our change is complete..... the day we put off this body of mortality and receive a new body of immortality. Then the struggle will be over! We will be free! And our change will finally be complete.

When our Heavenly Father, our Creator, looks at you, does He see a transformation taking place? A new you in the making? A woman with a new heart, changing day by day into a spiritual butterfly?

The next time you see a butterfly. Remember the One who created it. Remember His power of transformation and let Him work in you, day by day. Remind someone else of the transforming power of God.

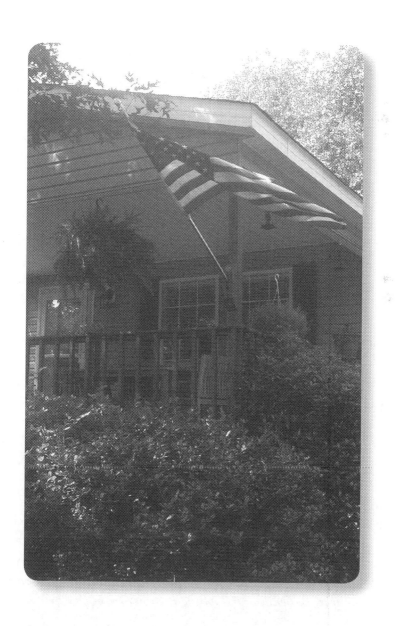

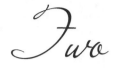

WIND

I love to watch our flag blowing in the wind and to hear the wind chimes, but I may need to take them down for a while. There is a storm coming in and the wind is up. I'm sitting on my front porch, watching and listening to the thunder a way off, coming closer and closer. Mr. Bluebird found a secure place to watch over his house and family. A hummingbird found a safe place to perch on my porch and we are watching the wind bring in a storm and I remember....... When my granddaughter, Adie, was as very little girl and the wind would start blowing, signaling a coming storm, she would run across the drive way and bang on my front door. "It's me! Let me in!" She was too little to open the door so I would let her in and she would go straight through the house to the back deck, and on her way, she will call out "get the cap..pu...chi...no!" and we would set on the back deck, watch the wind bring in the storm and enjoy cappuccino and each other.

And now, as I sit here and watch the wind blow through the trees, ruffle the flag and make the chimes ring, I remember Adie, and I remember what King David said, ***"God brings the wind out of His treasures".*** (Psalm 135:7)

Isn't that a lovely thought? Can you picture a large treasure chest in heaven holding all of God's treasures? And when the hand of the Almighty God lifts the lid, the wind is once again released for a time. But while it is free, Jesus said *"**The wind blows where it wishes, and you can hear the sound of it, but cannot tell where it comes from and where it goes.**"* (John 3:8)

But for all the freedom God gave the wind, He still uses it for His purposes. After God created His beautiful world, it gradually became so wicked, God decided to destroy it with water and that is the story of Noah and the ark. When the rain stopped, *He caused a wind to pass over the earth, and the waters subsided.* (Genesis 8:1)

When Moses brought the children of Israel out of Egypt and they were on their way back home, they came to the Red Sea. When they looked behind them, there was the Egyptian army coming after them! The sea in front and the enemy behind, with no way to escape! *The Lord caused the sea to go back by a strong east wind all that night and made the sea into dry land, and the waters divided.* (Exodus 14:21)

After the children of Israel had crossed the sea and were once again on their way, they faced a long journey. In time, they ran out of food and God used a wind to bring quail to feed His people. (Numbers 11:31)

God used the wind again when the prophet, Elijah had angered Queen Jezebel and she vowed to kill him. Elijah ran for his life and was hiding in a cave when the Lord came to reassure him that he was not alone and to remind him of Who was really in control. *God told him to "Go out and stand on the mountain before the Lord" and behold, the Lord passed by, and a great and strong wind tore into the mountains and broke the rocks in pieces before the Lord.* (1 Kings 19:11) How big a wind was that? Do you think Elijah got the message about who was really in control?

And with all it's freedom, Jesus still commands and controls the wind. Jesus and His disciples were crossing the Sea of Galilee when a great storm came up. Waves were filling the boat and Jesus was sleeping. When the men woke Him, He got up and rebuked the sea, *"Peace be still!" And the wind and the waves ceased and there was a great calm.* (Mark 4:35-39) Do you think they got the message? God, Christ, has all power over every thing! Even the wind.

Luke tells us the church was ushered in by *a sound from heaven, as of a rustling mighty wind and it filled the whole house.* It brought the Holy Spirit and filled those present with the ability to go out and teach every man in his own language. (Acts 2:1-12)

A strong wind destroyed the house where Job's children were all gathered for a meal. (Job 1:19) We can see the destructive forces a strong wind, a hurricane or a tornado can bring; property damage, power outages, even loss of life. But what does the wind look like in our lives?

Solomon says *"False boasting is like clouds and the wind without the rain."* (Proverbs 25:14) Ask a farmer how much good a hot dry wind does his crops. Useless!

Bildad asked his friend Job, *"How long are the words of your mouth going to be like a strong wind?"* (Job 82) Have you ever heard the expression, "That man sure is windy"? Annoying!

If you take an empty jar, go outside into a strong wind and let it blow into that empty jar and then clamp the lid on tight, what have you captured? Solomon tells us, laboring for riches is like laboring for the wind, for we cannot take riches into heaven. (Ecclesiastes 5:13-16) In eternity, a jar full of riches is like a jar full of wind! Empty!

Solomon also warns against causing friction in your home. If you bring anger, selfishness, animosity, etc. into your home, you will inherit the wind. (Proverbs 11:29) Unintended consequences of unhappiness will be the result.

Paul said *"we should no longer be children tossed to and fro and carried about with every wind of doctrine,"* easily deceived. (Ephesians 4:14)

James also warns, if we lack faith we will be tossed around by winds of doubt. (James 1:6) Having no understanding to our lives.

How can we avoid the winds of such devastation?

Jesus told a parable about a man who built his house on a rock and the winds came and beat on that house, but it did not fall. (Matthew 7:24-27) And that Rock was? Jesus Christ.

If Jesus can calm the wind that is capable of physical destruction, don't you think He can help you control the winds of anger, doubt, fear, false teaching and all the other howling winds that are blowing around inside you?

The next time the wind blows through your trees, ruffles your flag and rings your chimes, let it remind you; that, just as God is in control of the natural wind, He can help you... if you let Him... control those winds in your life.

Remind others of the power of God to control the wind in the trees and in their lives.

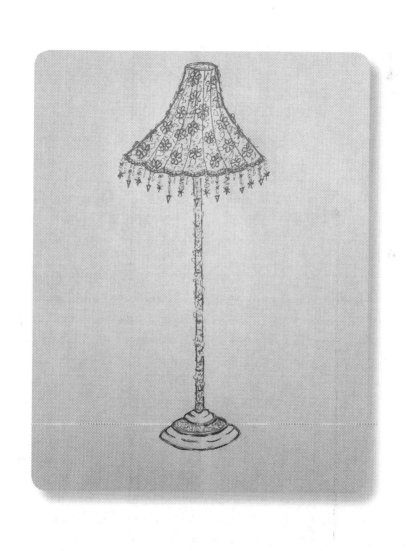

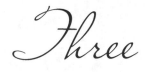

LIGHTS

When I was a little girl, my great grandmother had a floor lamp in her front parlor that was a work of art! It had colored glass jewels around the base and up the pole. The shade was covered with embroidered bead work and a fringe of beads hung from the scalloped edge. When you pulled the little gold chain, the lights made the jewels dance and sparkle. I thought it was the prettiest light anyone could ever see....until....the first year we were in Idaho.

My sister and I were already in bed asleep when our folks woke us up. We put our jackets on, got the lawn chairs and set down in the middle of the road, along with all the neighbors. We watched the Aurora Borealis for the first time! Talk about beautiful, dancing, colorful light! A whole sky full! My grandmother's lamp was no more the most beautiful light I had ever seen.

My sister and I shared a bedroom when we were little girls and Mother and Daddy put reflective decals on our ceiling. When we turned off our light at night, there, above our heads was the solar system! Daddy would lay on the floor with us and tell us all about the stars. He would show us the patterns and pictures they made and tell us their names.

Years later, floating down the Colorado River at one o'clock in the morning, I saw the Milky Way. It looked so close you could almost reach up into it, and I remembered that bedroom ceiling of so long ago. Did you know, God knows the name of each of those stars? (Psalm 147:4, Isaiah 40:22-26)

One of my favorite verses in the Bible was written by James, the brother of Jesus. ***Every good and perfect gift is from above, and it comes down*** *from the Father of Lights.* (James 1:17) Why did James call God the Father of Light?

God was creating the universe a*nd then God said "Let there be light" and there was light. And God saw the light that it was good. And God divided the light from the darkness.* A few verse down we read, *He said "Let there be lights in the firmament of heavens to give light on the earth." and it was so. Then God made two great lights: the greater light to rule the day and the lesser light to rule the night. He made the stars also.* (Genesis 1:3-4, 14-16)

Because God created humans with intelligence, it wasn't long before we realized light produces heat and energy, and the rest is history. Cooking fires, candles, oil lamps, electricity and who knows what the future holds? But it all started with the voice of God!

God is also the Father of another kind of light. All through scripture, light represents goodness, cleanness, honesty, knowledge and wisdom. We are also told light provides opportunities to produce these qualities.

The prophet, Zephaniah tells us light exposes complacency and brings justice. (Zephaniah 1:12)

David said *"You are a lamp, Oh Lord: The Lord shall enlighten my darkness"* (2 Samuel 22:29)

David also said, *"Your word is a lamp to my feet And a light to my path."* (Psalms 119:105)

Solomon tells us our conscience is the lamp of God. (Proverbs 20:27)

Daniel said of God, *"He reveals deep and secret things; He knows what is in the darkness and light dwells with Him."* (Daniel 2:22)

With His voice, God spoke physical light into existence. And with His word, His light; He teaches us, enlightens us, guides us and brings us out of spiritual darkness.

When Luke was writing the account of the birth of Jesus, he wrote down a prophecy made by Isaiah quoting God, referring to the coming of Christ. God said, *"I the Lord have called You in righteousness, And will hold your hand: I will keep You and give You as a covenant to the people and a light to the Gentiles."* (Isaiah 42:6, Luke 2:32)

The apostle John wrote, *In the beginning was the Word, and the Word was with God and the Word was God. He was in the beginning with God. In Him was life and the life was the light of men.* (John 1:1-4)

Jesus, Himself said, *"I am the light of the world. He who follows Me shall not walk in darkness but have the light of life."* (John 8:12)

God's Word is His Light, and that Light took on the form of man and came to walk on the earth. God's light was dressed as a man and we are to follow Him, walk in His light.

Have you ever been out on a dark, moonless, overcast night? Were you walking down a winding dirt road under a canopy of trees, a road you have never been on before? I have. You talk about dark! No way can you see the dangers before you. No way can you see the beauty around you. What to do? Turn your flashlight on, of course, and walk in the light it provides! If you are smart, you won't drop it by the side of the road or throw it into the ditch and go on without it. You will hang onto it and use it to guide you. It will show you the dangers and the beauty.

Jesus is the light in this world. What would the world be like without Him? He is the only source of light, of good. If people admit it or not, every bit of truth, mercy and love found even in the worst of us, comes from Christ!

But Jesus has returned to Heaven! Is the Light still here?

Jesus told His disciples, *"You are the light of the world....Let your light so shine before men that they may see your good works and glorify your Father in heaven."* (Matthew 5:14-16) About thirty years after Jesus returned to heaven, the apostle Paul wrote to the Christians in Ephesus, *For you were once in darkness, but now you are the light of the Lord. Walk as children of Light.* (Ephesians 5:8)

Before the days of the railroad, Americans had the Pony Express to deliver the mail across our vast country. Horse back riders were trained to carry the mail bag from one outpost to the next, where another man would take the bag and carry it to the next outpost. It was patterned after the Olympic games and the relay race, where a runner would carry a flaming torch and run his course, then pass the flame to the next runner who would run his assigned course.

Many times in his writing, the apostle Paul described a Christian life as running a race. He talked about endurance and self control while running this race. (1 Corinthians 9:24) He talked about running with certainty and assurance of direction. (Corinthians 9:26) He talked about being careful where you run. (Galatians 2:2) And he talked about holding on to the truth while you run. (Philippians 2:16)

Paul carried the torch, the light, through his life and he passed it on to Priscilla and Aquilla, Timothy, Titus and Philemon among many others. He taught them how to be the light and run their race, and he told them to tell others. Toward the end of his life, Paul said *"I have fought a good fight. I have finished the race, I have kept the faith."* (2 Timothy 4:7) And for almost two thousand years. that same light has been passed from one carrier to the next, to the next, to the next.

The answer to our question is YES! The light is still here.

You. Me. We are the light in this world! Christians are the light in this world. How is the light in your house? Is it growing dim or shinning brighter every day? Is your neighborhood growing darker or it brighter because of you?

Everyday, someone... your children, your neighbors, your co-workers... someone remarks about the weather. "The sun is really bright today." or "Did you see how bright the moon was last night?" Maybe they know about your grandmothers beautiful lamp. But do they know about the One True Light? Have they forgotten? *Should you remind them of the Father of Lights?*

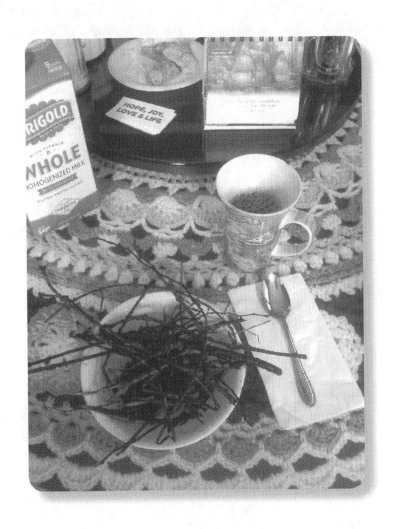

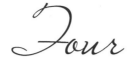

Four

STICKS AND TWIGS

When my children and grandchildren were growing up, I didn't keep a lot of junk cereal in the house. We "fixed" breakfast. I kept a box of "healthy" cereal for those days when I was by myself.

When she was little, my granddaughter, Katie spent the night with me and we had big plans for the next day. We were in a hurry so we had bowls of my healthy cereal. She turned her little nose up, but being a sweet little girl, she ate it....hesitantly, with a lot of facial expression, but no comments. And we were on our way.

Thereafter, whenever she was at my house at breakfast time, this question: "Nana, we aren't having sticks and twigs again, are we?"

Bread, food, meals, fun, family, friends, church family and sometimes, strangers! One word leads to another and eventually to good times and memories.

The Bible has a lot to say about food, and it is first mentioned at the very beginning. God provided everything Adam and Eve could possibly eat for a balanced diet. Talking to Adam, ***God said, "Have dominion over the fish of the sea, over the birds of the air, and over every living thing that moves on the earth. I have given you every herb that yields seed which is on the earth, and every tree whose fruit yields seed; for you it shall be for food,"*** (Genesis 1:28-29) After Adam and Eve left the garden, we are told their sons became herdsmen and farmers. (Genesis 4:1-2)

When the children of Israel were wandering in the wilderness, The Lord God supplied them with meat every evening and bread every morning. (Exodus 16:12-15) Here it is called bread, in verse 31 it was called Manna and later on Moses gives us a more complete description and more ways to prepare it. (Numbers 11) The word "Manna" means "what is it?" No one had ever seen it before and they didn't have a name for it. We would have called it "what- ch- ma- call- it". They could grind it into flour for bread. They could add honey and bake cakes, boil it, rather like cream of wheat cereal. How ever they prepared it, God supplied a daily ration for each of them.

God used ravens to brings bread and meat to Elijah during a time of drought. (1 Kings 17:1-6)

Another story about food. The book of Ruth is a story about a young woman who was born and raised in the idol worshiping country of Moab. She married into a family of foreigners from Judah. In time, her father-in-law, her brother-in-law and her husband all died. Her mother-in-law, Naomi, decided to go back home and she instructed her two daughters-in-law to go back to their families. One of the women did, but Ruth had learned to love Naomi and made the decision to go with her. Ruth's beautiful statement of commitment has been recorded for us. Two beautiful verses of love and devotion. (Ruth1:16-17) The rest of the story tells of the love and compassion Ruth had for Naomi and the love and compassion Boaz, the owner of commercial grain fields, had for the young woman, Ruth. Because there were no men in the family to care for the two women, Boaz gave Ruth a protected position so she could work in safety for food for her beloved Naomi. By the way, this isn't the end of Ruth's story. The life of Jesus is the end of Ruth's story. She became the grandmother of King David, from whose family Jesus is descended.

We are told of at least two times that Jesus was welcomed into the home of Mary of Bethany for meals, once when He and His apostles came through her town on their travels, (Luke 10:38) and again she entertained Him, just six days before His Crucifixion. (John 12:1-2)

Several times, Jesus fed others. Once the disciples came in from a fishing trip and Jesus had a campfire going and a breakfast of fish and bread (the first fish sandwich, maybe?) ready for them when they came ashore. (John 21:3-9)

Multitudes followed Jesus every where He went and more than once He fed them all. Matthew tells us of an evening when Jesus fed five thousand men plus women and children! Possibly up to twelve thousand or more hungry mouths at one time! (Matthew 14:13-21)

Jesus fed the hungry and He instructed us and set us the example of feeding the hungry. He said when we feed and care for the poor and hungry, we are taking care of Him. *"In as much as you did it to the least of these, You did it to Me."* (Matthew 25:31-46)

The apostles Paul and James tell us, not only are we to work for our own food, but we are to work to help the needy, the widows and orphans. (Ephesians 4:28, James 1:27)

Jesus also taught there is more than one kind of food. There is physical food and there is spiritual food. After Jesus was baptized by John, He went into the wilderness and after forty days of fasting, the tempter (the devil, Satan) came and said to Him *"If you are the Son of God, command that these stones become bread" but He answered and said "It is written, Man shall not live by bread alone, but by every word that proceeds out of the mouth of God."* (Matthew 4:3-4)

The apostle John tells us that in the beginning the **Word was with God and the Word was God.** (John 1:1-5) Later, John records Jesus as saying *"I am the bread of life. He who comes to Me shall never hunger."* (John 6:35) So, the words of Jesus are the words of God and they are our spiritual bread. Later, John tell us why he recorded the words of Jesus. *These things I have written to you who believe in the name of the Son of God, that you may know you have eternal life and that you may continue to believe in the name of the Son of God.* (1 John 5:13) The bread of Life, the words of Jesus, have been preserved for us so we can feed on His words, study, increase our faith and have eternal life.

Jesus taught us, there is still yet, another kind of bread. For us to understand this kind of bread, we need to back up for a short history lesson.

When the children of Israel were slaves in Egypt, Moses brought a message from the Lord to Pharaoh, and because Pharaoh would not listen to the message, God delivered nine terrible plagues on Egypt, trying to convince Pharaoh to let his people go, but Pharaoh steadfastly refused. (Exodus chapters 7-10) Now God was going to bring one last plague. The Death Angel was coming to take the first born of every woman and animal. (Exodus chapters 11 and 12) Moses also brought instructions from God to the children of Israel. The only way an Israelite family could escape this death was by killing a perfect, sacrificial lamb and putting the blood of the lamb on the doorpost of their house. They were to roast the meat and prepare a supper that included unleavened bread. This was the first Passover and it was to be celebrated every year thereafter as a reminder of

God's mercy and His saving power. Later, the people were taught that one day, a Messiah would come and another tradition began. Every year on the Passover table was an extra glass of wine in expectation that one day the Messiah would join them for the Passover meal. But this is just the beginning of the story.

Fourteen hundred and fifty years later, when Jesus was celebrating the feast of the Passover with His disciples, He explained the rest of the story. After all these years, no longer would a sacrificial Passover lamb be necessary, or the blood of that lamb. Never again! In just a few hours, He would become the last, the final sacrificial lamb! And that glass of wine? It would now represent His blood that would be shed. That unleavened bread that was prepared every year? Now it would become the symbol of His body that was to be sacrificed! Not generations later, not years later, but the next day! (Matthew 26:17-29)

The apostle Paul wrote that Jesus gave him instructions to pass on to the church concerning that last meal that Jesus had. ***Jesus, on the same night in which He was betrayed, took bread and when He had given thanks, He broke it and said "Take eat, this is My body. Do this in remembrance of Me." He also took the cup and said "This cup is the new covenant in my blood. This do, as often as you drink it, in remembrance of Me."*** (1 Corinthians 11:23-26)

Luke wrote, ***Now on the first day of the week, when the disciples came together to break bread, Paul ready to depart on the next day, spoke to them and continued his message until midnight.*** (Acts 20:7)

Their purpose for coming together was to break the bread in remembrance of Jesus and His sacrificial death and His resurrection that took place on that wonderful Sunday morning. And so we do, every Sunday. We celebrate this feast in remembrance of the last Sacrificial Lamb. We are no longer commanded to keep Passover once a year, to remember the release of the children out of Egyptian bondage, as under the old covenant. Now, under the new covenant, we remember every first day of the week, our release from the bondage of sin.

So....the next time you have a bowl of "Sticks and Twigs" (or Cheerios); or you study your Bible, the bread of life; or you participate in the Lord's supper, remember....your physical food, your spiritual food and your memorial food, all come from the One True God, the Great Provider.

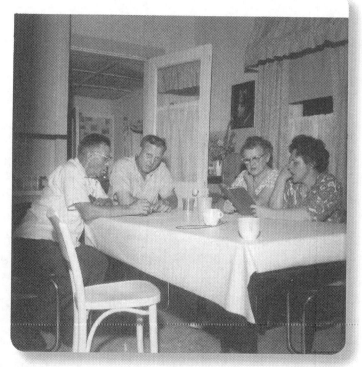

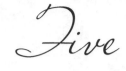

SINGING

When I think about singing, the first thing that comes to mind is my grandmother's kitchen table and my folks singing songs from the church hymnal. My grandfather and my dad were song leaders and I think they wanted to know every song in the book. One of my most treasured photographs was taken of them around that table.

When we visit the nursing home, many of those residents are struggling with memory loss. But, when we sing the old hymns, their eyes light up. They remember! And they sing out. Many don't remember who I am or what they had for lunch, but they remember singing to God!

The Bible has a lot to say about singing. It tells us all nature sings the glory of it's Creator. King David spoke of birds singing. ***The birds of the heavens have their habitation. They sing among the branches.*** (Psalms 104:12)

The mountains and the hills shall break forth into singing before the Lord (Isaiah 55:12)

The trees of the woods shall rejoice before the Lord (1 chronicles 16:33)

All of you have heard the birds singing. How many of you have been in the mountains and heard the wind whistling through the pine trees? These are some of God's beautiful songs.

God told Job the morning stars sing together. (Job 38:7) Researchers have recorded sounds from outer space, musical chords. And there is nothing out there but stars!

The first song recorded in scripture was sung by Moses and the Israelites after their release from Egyptian bondage. A wonderful song praising God for His triumphal deliverance, His glorious power and the greatness of His excellence. It was a way to remember all God had done for them. (Exodus 15)

The magnificent song of Mary, preserved for us by Luke, is truly a song we can sing today. It is a song of praise sung from her soul, magnifying her God, her Savior. She recognized the blessings God had given her and those who were yet to come. She sings of the mercy He shows to His people, through all generations. She sings of His strength and power to punish and reward. She sings of His care for the poor and how He spoke words to Abraham that would be for all of Abraham's spiritual family (the Christian family) forever. (Luke 1:46-55)

Jesus and His twelve apostles sang a hymn together after they shared the Lord's supper. (Mark 14:26) I've often wondered which hymn they sang. Wouldn't you love to have heard their voices? This was to be the last song they would sing together, for Jesus would be arrested that same night and put to death the next day. Do you think that song was special to each of them? I wonder how many times they would sing it in years to come and remember their Friend and Savior?

Luke tells us Paul and Silas were praying and singing while in prison waiting for their trial! (Acts 16:25) These two men had been beaten, put into the "inner prison" (dungeon) and put in chains. They were facing a trial that could end in their execution and they were singing hymns and praying! How many others in that same position would be screaming and cursing God?

Have your burdens ever been so heavy, your mind so troubled, you couldn't form a prayer, but a song just kept running through your head? Or you couldn't put the words together to form a prayer of your own. There were just no words to say how you were feeling. I pray a lot of King David's prayers. I sing a lot of his songs. I wish I knew what songs Paul and Silas were singing to give themselves courage, strength and to keep their faith strong. Maybe they sang these Psalms:

Hear me when I call, O God of my righteousness! You have relieved me when I was in distress; Have mercy on me, and hear my prayer. (Psalm 4:1)

The Lord is my strength and my shield. My heart trusted in Him and I am helped, Therefore my heart greatly rejoices, And with my song I will praise Him! (Psalms 28:7)

God is our refuge and strength, A very present help in the time of trouble. Therefore we will not fear. (Psalms 46:1)

Let all those rejoice who put their trust in You! Let them ever shout for joy, because You defend them. Let those who love Your name be joyful in You! (Psalms 5:11-12)

James tells us to sing Psalms when we are happy (James 5:13) How about singing these Psalms:

Let the righteous be glad, Let them rejoice before God; Yes, let them rejoice exceedingly! Sing to God, sing praises to His name; Extol Him who rides on the clouds, By His name YAH, and rejoice before Him. (Psalms 68:3-4)

I will praise you, O Lord, with my whole heart. I will tell of Your marvelous works. I will be glad and rejoice in You. I will sing praises to Your name, O Most High! (Psalms 9:1-2)

Make a joyful noise before the Lord, all you lands! Serve the Lord with gladness. Come before His presence with singing. (Psalms 100:1-2)

Paul wrote to the church in Corinth and told them to sing with the spirit and with the understanding. (1 Corinthians 14:15) He told the church in Colossae to teach and encourage one another with singing. (Colossians 3:16) There is a congregation that built a new building and one thing they requested of the architect was to design an auditorium where all in attendance could look across and face other worshipers. The reason for this request? So each member could sing, not only praises to God, but encouragement and words of wisdom to one another.

One of my favorite verses in the Bible is found in Zephaniah 3:17. *The Lord your God is in your midst, the Almighty One will save. He will rejoice over you with gladness. He will quiet you in His love. He will rejoice over you with singing.*

Your God sings over you! Let that sink in a minute. The Lord, God Almighty sings over you!

We sing "Happy Birthday over people to celebrate with them. We sing lullabies over our infants and "Jesus loves me" over our children. We sing at funerals to bring comfort to those in mourning. We sing the "Twenty Third Psalm" to encourage them. If you love someone, sing over them.

Sing with them, teach them the songs. Let others hear you sing. One of the best gifts you can give your children and grandchildren is to let them hear you singing Psalms and hymns and praying around the house. They don't care if you are a little off key. They hear you expressing love for their Father in heaven.

Sing to remind yourself, how much God loves you. Sing over others to remind them. Go outside and join in with God's creation and sing a song from your soul, like Mary, and thank Him for all he has done and continues to do.

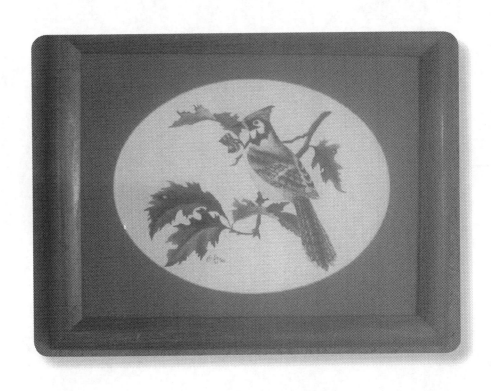

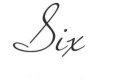

BIRDS

Most mornings we spend time on the front porch. My husband Mike, me, the binoculars and the coffee pot. We live in a perfect place to watch birds. There are geese and ducks on the pond, occasionally a great blue heron and all kinds of birds come to the feeders. We found woodpeckers to be easy going. Blue Jays are bullies! All the rest fall somewhere in between, depending on the season and Hummingbirds only fight among themselves. There is a pair of bluebirds that raise two broods in our box every year. They all entertain us and we miss those that don't show up for breakfast.

All through the centuries, birds have been the subject of folk lore, traditions and superstitions. They are the universal symbol of freedom; they can walk, swim, hop and fly. They each have their own suit of clothes and their own song. Birds are believed to be the herald of birth, the sign of the seasons, the messengers of joy and the omen of death. A flock of Hummingbirds is called a "charm" and a flock of ravens is called an "unkindness". Cardinals are said to represent nobility. Chickadees symbolize purity. Blue Birds bring happiness. Owls represent wisdom and Canaries are the sign of joy.

Since ancient times, Birds have been kept for pets because of their beauty, their song and their ability to mimic. My aunt had a parakeet named Peaty. His perch was across the room from the front door and everyone that came in was greeted with "Hello Beautiful" and when they left, it was "Bye Baldy"

Birds have always been used for food. King David called quail, bread of heaven (Psalms 105:40) referring to God's provision for the children of

Israel in the wilderness when He sent quail every evening to provide meat for them. (Exodus 16:13)

Samuel, the prophet, mentions hunting partridge for food. (1 Samuel 26:20)

There are fifty-five verses in the Bible using birds to convey messages of hope, strength, destruction and deliverance.

When the dove was released from the ark and she returned with an olive leaf, it was a sign that the flood was receding. When she was released again and didn't return, Noah knew it would soon be time to leave the ark. (Genesis 8:8-12)

A dove was the Father's sign of approval at the baptism of His Son. *And Jesus saw the Spirit of God descending like a dove and alighting upon Him. And suddenly a voice from heaven saying "This is My Son, in whom I am well pleased."* (Matthew 3:17)

When Jesus was teaching a lesson on how His apostles were to conduct themselves as they walked through this world delivering His message, *He said "Behold, I send you out as sheep in the midst of wolves. Therefore be wise as serpents and harmless as doves."* (Matthew 10:16-18) Now that you are followers of Me, He said, and carrying My message, be aware, there are those in the world who will attack you and the message. Be smart, prepare yourselves, be ready for trouble, but always carry the message with humbleness and love.

God reminded His children how He delivered them out of Egypt: *"and how I bore you on eagles' wings and brought you to Myself."* (Exodus 19:4)

Have you ever had the opportunity to watch eagles? When a storm is moving in, they go up, up, up above the storm and wait it out.

Isaiah tells us *Those that wait on the Lord shall renew their strength; they shall mount up with wings like eagles. They shall run and not be weary, they shall walk and not faint.* (Isaiah 40:31) Eagles don't go head first into a storm and fight through it. They rise about it, conserve their strength and so are able to continue on for long distances.

Each one of us will have spiritual storms, emotional storms, physical storms in our lives. Decisions to make about right and wrong, disagreements with family or friends, problems at work, sickness, disabilities, even death. A lot of these storms can be prevented, avoided or mitigated......or made worse. How many storms do we cause? How many times do we join in a storm and make it worse or keep it going? Maybe we should have just left.

If we let Him, Jesus can show us how to live our lives without a storm every day. He doesn't want us to live "soap-opera" lives. When storms do come, and they will, don't let your anxiety, anger or your sorrow guide you. You do not have to be defeated or destroyed by a storm. You can rise above it. Some, you need to avoid all together! Admit to yourself, you need God's help. Then let Him help you! ***I can do all things through Christ who strengthens me.*** (Philippians 4:13)

Jesus used a sparrow to demonstrate that God, our Father is aware of each of us and our needs, and He values us more than the sparrows. ***"Are not two sparrows sold for a copper coin? And not one of them falls to the ground apart from your Father's will. But the very hairs on your head are numbered. Do not fear therefore; you are of more value than many sparrows"*** (Matthew 10:29-31)

When Jesus was lamenting over the city of Jerusalem, because of the unwillingness of the spiritual leaders and civic leaders to accept Him, He said: ***"Oh Jerusalem, Jerusalem, the one who kills the prophets and stones those who are sent to her! How often I wanted to gather your children together as a hen gathers her chicks under her wings, but you were not willing."*** (Matthew 23:37) Most of the people just would not listen to Jesus. He wanted them to have better lives. He could have helped them have better lives. He wanted to protect them from many of the problems and sorrows in this life and keep them from spiritual death in the next. But they would not let Him! Have you ever watched a hen protect her eggs in her nest or her baby chicks. She can be really aggressive!! Jesus did everything He could to get them to listen to Him. He taught them. He fed them. He healed them. He even raised their dead for them! He begged them; listen to Me!! I can help you!! But they would not.

God used all these wonderful, beautiful birds to show us His love and concern; to teach us how to live better lives, lives that look like Jesus. Then He shows us a bird that is the perfect example of what not to be. He used an ostrich.... to show us what the lack of wisdom looks like: harsh, wasteful, vain, no understanding. (Job 39:13-18)

My prayer for you is that you may be gentle as a dove, rise about your problems on wings of eagles, allow Jesus to protect you as a hen protects her chicks and NEVER BE AN OSTRICH.

Whenever you see or hear a bird, take a minute to admire it's beauty and it's song. And remember it's Maker, it's Protector and it's Provider. And remember...He will provide all these things for you too...if you will let Him. And if someone else is with you, remind them, about the birds of the Bible and their stories.

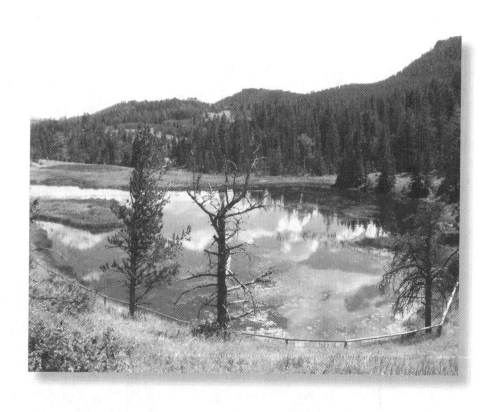

Seven

MIRRORS

When my sister was a little girl, I found her standing on a step stool looking into the bathroom mirror with tears running down her face. I asked her what in the world was wrong!? "I'm trying to make a scary face and I just look funny!" Lesson learned........a mirror reflects what is put into it!

We've only had mirrors, as we know them, since 1835. A German chemist invented the process of applying a thin layer of silver to the back of clear glass. Before that, people used polished stone, such as obsidian to see their reflection. Before that, mirrors were made from polished bronze, silver or brass.

In the book of Genesis we read about Cain's descendent, Tubal-Cain, receiving the God-given ability to make things from metal. Maybe he made the first metal mirrors. (Genesis 4:22)

The first time a mirror is mentioned in scripture is found in the book of Job. Most Bible scholars think Job lived sometime around or just before Abraham, so his story should fall, chronologically somewhere around Genesis, chapter eleven or twelve, but it wasn't written until later. It was Job's friend, Elihu, who mentioned a "cast" (hot metal poured into shaped molds specificity made for that purpose) metal mirror. (Job 37:18)

Have you ever stepped to the edge of a lake and observed your own reflection in the water? If you stand back, you can see the refection of the opposite shore replicated perfectly. Or you can look across the surface and see the sky. Did you know, it is the refection of the blue sky that makes the lake water look blue? On a cloudy day, that same water will look gray. Or maybe it will reflect the forest along the shore and look green. Water has no color of it's own; like a mirror, it only reflects what is put into it.

King Solomon said, *as it is with water, face reveals face, so a man's heart reveals the man.* (Proverbs 27:19) you reflect what is in your heart. Jesus said, *Out of the abundance of the heart, the mouth speaks.* (Matthew 12:34) Your mouth is the reflection of your heart, which is a reflection of you.

King David said, *I will see Your face in righteousness; I shall be satisfied when I awake in your likeness.* (Psalms 17:15) He said he would see the refection of the Lord in the right living of others, but he would really be happy when he woke up from death and looked like the Lord!

The apostle Paul wrote *But we all with unveiled face, beholding as in a mirror the glory of the Lord, are being transformed into the same image.* (2 Corinthians 3:18) With unveiled face means with no self deception; open honesty. When we see ourselves as we really are, only then can we begin our transformation until we look into the mirror and see Him!

You've heard that old saying "like mother, like daughter". It means you act like your mother! People see her in you. You learned from her. You do things the way she did. You use her recipes. You have the same expressions, the same temperament; you mirror or reflect your mother. Maybe you reflect your dad or an aunt, maybe a teacher. If you know your mother's name, but you never knew her. Maybe you heard others talk about her, but you never spent time with her, how much like her would you be?

You may think you are a reflection of Christ because you have heard of Him, heard others speak of Him. Maybe you heard a preacher, or a friend speak of Him, but have you spent time with Him? Listened to Him? Have you picked up His habits of doing good; helping and teaching others, loving and forgiving others? Do you really reflect Christ? Did you learn from Him? Do you say things like Him? Do you have His temperament, His attitude? You can't reflect Christ until you know Him. The more you know Him, the more you will look like Him, sound like Him, act like Him.

Remember the lake we were talking about? When the wind is calm, the water gives a perfect reflection of you. If the wind is up, it will cause ripples which damage your reflection. If a storm blows in, it can remove all traces of your reflection.

Are you giving a clear reflection of Jesus or a distorted one? How clear is His image when small disturbances damage your reflection of Him? How much of Jesus do others see in you when a major problem arises? Do you loose your reflection of Jesus completely?

Sometimes a mirror can have flaws, and an imperfect mirror will give off an imperfect reflection.

Have you ever been to a house of mirrors? The mirrors are intentionally giving a false reflection. We can look very elongated or very short, extremely thin or heavy, our arms too short, our heads too big. A very bad reflection! If you claim to be a Christian, but the image you give doesn't look like Christ, maybe you need to get busy and readjust your mirror.

Sometimes a mirror may become dirty. Maybe over time it has developed a cloudy look or the silver back may become damaged. Does that mirror reflect the image you want it to, or do you need to spend some time cleaning it again or making some repairs? Do you need to spend more time with Jesus? Learn from Him again? You are a mirror and you are constantly giving off a reflection, whether you want to not. What do others see when they look at you? Do they see a clear, clean reflection of Jesus?

I have no idea who first wrote this, but I copied it and taped it to my bathroom mirror: "If I could look into this mirror and see my character instead of my face, what would I see" This is my way of reminding myself everyday, sometimes several times a day, to pray King David's prayer ***Create in me a new heart, O God and renew a steadfast spirit within me.*** (Psalms 51:10) The heart, the mind is where the reflection comes from. It isn't the reflection of your face that is important to your Heavenly Father! What does your heart look like?

In this life, on this earth, we will never look exactly like our Lord, but He can help us fix our flaws and repair our hearts so we can cast a more perfect reflection. And He will help us look better day by day, so those around us can see Him more clearly and be reminded of "The Man" who loved, provided for, protected, taught and forgave those around Him.

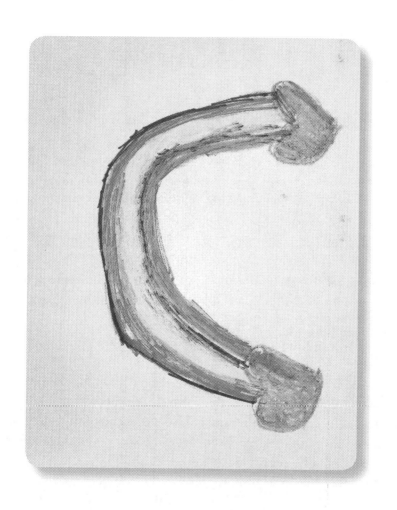

RAINBOWS

One of the first things a child learns to do with crayons is to draw stick figures of Mom and Daddy, Grandma, a house, maybe the family cat or dog. But the next picture is usually a rainbow. There is something magical about the combination of the perfect arch and just the right colors and try as we might, no one comes close to God's rainbows. But we have tried all through the centuries because the mystery of the rainbow is intriguing.

Some Australian Aborigine tribes believe in the "rainbow serpent" as the creator.

The belief that the rainbow is a bridge that connect the realm of gods and humans is found in many cultures; Japan, India and Greece among others.

Hawaiian myth says the rainbow transports the souls of the dead to paradise.

Some Arabians and some African people believe the rainbow is used by the thunder god to send down arrows of destruction.

The Irish believe there is a pot of gold at the end of the rainbow. How many stories and movies have been made about rainbows and leprechauns guarding a pot of gold?

A whole generation of kids grew up singing "Somewhere Over the Rainbow" and kids in our Bible classes sing "Blue Skies and Rainbows and Sunbeams from Heaven"

A favorite childhood story is the biblical account of Noah and the flood. Children love the story about the ark, all the animals and the first rainbow. As we grow older, we understand the deeper story of God's love, mercy and saving power found in that story, but the rainbow is what comes to mind first.

The rainbow is a story unto itself. It represents the promise God made to Noah. *"And it shall be, when I bring a cloud over the earth, that the rainbow shall be seen in the cloud and I will remember My covenant which is between Me and you and every living creature of all flesh; the water shall never again become a flood to destroy all flesh."* (Genesis 9:14-15) Did you get that? God made the rainbow to remind Himself of the agreement He made with Noah.

When you see a rainbow, do you remember God's promise? When you see a rainbow, do you think about God's power? The power only God has to bring about such destruction? Nothing is beyond the power of God and He has given us a thing of beauty to remind us not only of His power, but of His willingness to restrain that power.

While the earth remains, Seed time and harvest, And cold and heat, And winter and summer, And day and night shall not cease. (Genesis 8:22) Not only will the earth not be destroyed by water again, but as long as there is an earth, it will provide everything necessary to sustain life on it. In the beginning man was told to tend and care for the earth, (Genesis 2:15) but there is nothing we can do to bring it to an end or to make it continue. God is in control of that.

The Bible is full of promises made by God. Joshua reminded the children of Israel that God had kept every promise He had ever made! *"All of them have come to pass, and not one word of them has failed."* (Joshua 23:14) We are going to look at a few of those promises.

In his letter to the Ephesian church, Paul reminded them of the first commandment which held a promise. (Ephesians 6:2-3) That commandment and promise is the fifth of the ten commandments which God gave to Moses. *Honor your father on your mother that your days may be long* (Exodus 20:12) It doesn't say until you are eighteen or twenty one. It doesn't say until your parents die. It is unqualified. It means until you die!

God promised Abraham and Sarah a son (Genesis 18:10) And in time, Sarah gave birth to Isaac (Genesis 21:3)

God told Abraham, his descendants would be in bondage in a foreign land for four hundred years and then He promised they would return home. (Genesis 15:13-14) and that is the story of Moses. The book of Exodus tells us how he brought Abraham's family out of Egypt and led them across the wilderness. The book of Joshua tells us how he took the family into Canaan. Promise kept!

When Israel was facing the Midianites, God told Gideon, He would fight for him and Israel would win the battle. (Judges 7) God used a funny way to select an army for Gideon. Thirty two thousand men were eligible to serve, but God said that was too many. So the number was reduced to ten thousand, but God said that was still too many. God told Gideon to bring the men to the river and He would select the army by the way they drank water! Verse 7: Then the Lord said to Gideon, *"By the three hundred men who lapped I will save you and deliver the Midianites into your hand."* And verse 25 describes how the Midianites were defeated and everyone knew it was done by the power of God, not by a big army. Another promise kept!

God told Samuel He would destroy the house (family) of Eli because of sin and He did (1 Samuel 3:11-14, 1 Samuel 4:11)

God made a promise to the Israelites, *The days are coming* (when the time is right) *when I will make a new covenant"* this one will not be written on tables of stone but, *"I will put my laws in their minds and on their hearts"----* *"and their sin I will remember no more"* (Jeremiah 31:31-34) Unlike the old covenant, which required each person's sins to be remembered every year with a sacrifice and forgiven for one year at a time, but never completely forgiven; this new covenant would provide a way for all those past sins and all those committed in the future by unknown generations to be completely forgiven, to be remembered no more. What a promise that was!

All the prophets of the Old Testament told us about a time when things would change. A new law and a new teacher. No longer, Abraham or Moses but the Christ. Over three hundred God given prophesies concerning the coming of Christ and His new covenant are recorded in the Old Testament.

The apostle, Matthew records Jesus saying *"For this is My blood of the new covenant, which is shed for many for the forgiveness of sins"* (Matthew 26:28) Jesus brought the new covenant! *For God so loved the world that He gave His only begotten Son, that whosoever believes*

in Him should not perish but have everlasting life. (John 3:16) Jesus brought forgiveness of sins. Promise kept!

God promised Abraham that in (through) him, all the families of the earth shall be blessed, not just his family. (Genesis 12:3) God repeated this promise to Isaiah when He said the time would come when ***My house shall be called a house of prayer for all nations.*** (Isaiah 56:7) Promise made.

For thousands of years, God's family were the descendants of Abraham. Matthew (1:1-17) and Luke (3:23-38) both tell us Jesus was descended from that family. It was because of Him that all nations would be blessed, no longer just the Jewish nation. The first people who heard the gospel, responded through baptism and became followers of Jesus were Jews. (Acts 2) Then we read about Cornelius, a Gentile. (Acts 10) The Jewish people referred to anyone who was not a Jew as a Gentile. When Cornelius and his family heard the gospel, were baptized and became followers of Jesus, the promise came true! All families, all nations, all people could now be blessed by God! Promise kept!

There is yet another promise to be kept. Jesus said He would come again! He said there will come a time when the people of the earth would no longer believe in Him and His word and ***"all the tribes of the earth will mourn, and they will see the Son of Man coming on the clouds of heaven with power and great glory".*** (Matthew 24:30)

Jesus told His disciples ***"In My Father's house are many mansions, if it were not so, I would have told you. I go to prepare a place for you. And if I go to prepare for you, I will come again and receive you to myself, that where I am, you may be also."*** (John 14:2-3)

"And this is the will of Him who sent Me. That everyone who sees the Son and believes in Him may have everlasting life and I will raise him on that last day." (John 6:40)

The New Testament Christians were tired of waiting for Christ to come again. They were suffering because of their belief and wanted Jesus to come now! (2 Peter 8-10) They were getting impatient and the apostle Peter told them to be patient. With God a day is like a thousand years and a thousand years is as a day. Christ will come when God thinks the time is right. Don't give up. ***The Lord is not slack concerning His promise, as some count slackness, but is long suffering toward us, not willing that any should perish but that all should come to repentance.*** (verse

9) God is being patient with His creation. He doesn't want anyone one to perish! He wants everyone to come to repentance. But one day, He will grow tired of waiting.

Jesus said *"But of that day and hour, no one knows, no not even the angels of heaven, but My Father only."* And He went on to say some people will be looking for and preparing for Him, others won't *"Therefore, be ready, for the Son of Man is coming at an hour when you do not expect Him."* (Matthew 24:36, 44)

Do you think God will keep this last promise?

The rainbow is a reminder of promises made. The rain will end, and the sun will shine again. Life will continue on the earth. It may not always be just what we would like it to be, but if we allow Him, He can make it better. And if we co-operate with Him, He has promised an eventual perfection for each of us through His Son, Jesus Christ. Heaven! Now that is a promise I want to see fulfilled!

Next time a rain shower comes up, take your kids or your grand kids out side (a little bit of rain won't melt you and you can dry your hair later) and dance in the rain. Dance for the pure joy of it and look for the rainbow. Remind those children of God's promises made and kept. Promises made for them! They will never forget dancing in the rain with you. They will tell their children and grandchildren of the day they danced in the rain with you and looked for the rainbow. And they will tell of the promises kept and promises to come.

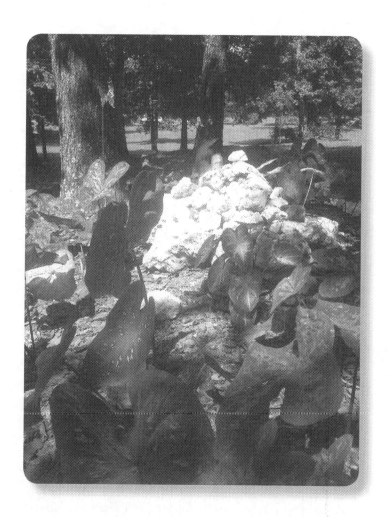

ROCKS

When my parents moved my grandparents, Mamo and Papo, across country from Ohio to Idaho, my grandmother took her rocks with her. Twenty years later they moved to Texas where I was living. They came with a big moving fan full of house hold items, dad's camper was packed full. The car was loaded and it had a little trailer behind it full of....you guessed it....Mamo's rocks.

She had rocks from every place she had ever been and more rocks from places she had never been! Friends and relatives would bring her rocks from their travels. She pained names, dates and places on each one. They were her way of remembering.

Dad learned to appreciate the beauty of rocks when we first moved to Idaho "The Gem State" and he became a rock hound extraordinaire. He was always searching for just the right rock to turn into beautiful jewelry; Opal, jasper, quartz and gold among others. He kept a bowl of wonderful tumbled rocks for the grand kids to play with and to give to anyone who wanted them. A lot of us still wear Dad's jewelery and we remember him when we do.

My youngest granddaughter, Gracy, learned the love of rocks from my dad, so when I went on a European journey, "Following the steps of Paul", I collected a small rock for her everywhere I went. I put each one in a small bag along with a note, where it came from and what Paul said or did in that place. Her mother had the rocks and notes put into a shadow box to hang on her wall.

When my husband Mike and I moved to Arkansas, we discovered chrystal rocks. What a treasure! When my granddaughters came for a visit, we went rock hunting and they collected so many they couldn't take all of them home. Even then, the car was "low riding" for sure. The extras were stacked in a cairn in my flower garden. Now, years later, when I walk past that pile of rocks, I remember, The Almighty Creator and my little rock hound.

When John described the holy city, New Jerusalem, the bride of Christ,(the church Jesus built) (Revelation 21:2), as he saw it in his vision, the new city was surrounded by a wall built of every precious stone; Jasper, sapphire, emerald beryl, amethyst among others. The gates were pearls and the streets were pure gold. (Revelation 21:18-21) What a beautiful place that is!

God created all these rocks, He used them and required men to use them for special purposes.

How many alters were built as places to worship the Creator? And God's instructions were ***"You shall not built it of hewn stone for if you use your tool on it, you have profaned it."*** (Exodus 20:25) God didn't want them cut to shape. They were perfect for His purpose just as they were.

Moses led the children of Israel out of Egypt and they were on their way to Canaan they traveled through a vast wilderness. By the time they arrived in Rephidim they had run out of water and there was no water there. But there was a rock. God told Moses to strike the rock and when he did, God used that rock to supply water for over two million people, all their flocks and all their herds. That was some rock! (Exodus 17:1-7)

Scientists thought they had discovered something new when they found they could extract oil from rocks. God told Moses how to do that over fourteen hundred years ago! (Deuteronomy 32:13)

When the Israelites walked on dry land through the river into the land of Canaan, God told Joshua to have twelve large stones stacked as a memorial to teach future generations about the miraculous crossing of the Jordan River. (Joshua 4:1-7)

The prophet Habakkuk recalled God's words concerning wicked men who built towns and cities and their own houses by evil means. They cheated people, didn't pay their debts, took advantage of people and spilled the blood of others. They were full of pride, covetous and they conducted their households shamefully. God said the day will come when the very stones used to build the walls will cry out against those men! (Habakkuk 2:9-11)

The Pharisees didn't like it when the people of Jerusalem were in the streets, welcoming Christ, celebrating, rejoicing and praising God for all His mighty works. When the Pharisees came to Christ and said "Rebuke these people! Tell them to stop!" Jesus replied *"I tell you that if these should be quiet, the stones would immediately cry out."*(Luke 19:37-40) The earth itself, God's creation, knows the Son of God and recognizes righteousness and goodness.

Job wanted his words *engraved on a rock With an iron pen and lead, forever! For I know my Redeemer lives, and He shall stand at last on the earth!* (Job 19:23-25) Job's faith was so strong and he knew his faith would not diminish! He wanted this powerful truth engraved in stone forever! Do you believe something to the point that you are willing to have it written in stone, never change your mind, never have second thoughts about it, forever remembered that you said it? How about on your tomb stone? Would you have a statement of your faith written there for all the world to see?

The Bible not only tells us God and men used rocks from God's creation for building and writing, but it also tells us of another kind of rock. The One, True Rock!

King David's words have been preserved for centuries. He proclaimed *The Lord is my rock and my fortress and my my deliverer.* (Psalms 18:2) *"The Lord lives! Blessed be the Rock! Let God be exalted! The Rock of my Salvation!"* (2 Samuel 22:47) *He only is my rock and my salvation, I shall not be moved!* (Psalms 62:2) David built his unshakeable faith on the Rock of salvation.

More than fourteen hundred years after Moses struck the rock and it brought water, Paul wrote to the Corinthian church and told them the story of Moses and the rock that gave water, then Paul said *That Rock was Christ* (1Corinthians 10:1-4) That rock in the wilderness, which gave physical water is the Rock which gives us spiritual water today.

Matthew records a parable of Jesus in which He said *"Therefore, whoever hears these words of Mine, and does them. I will liken him to a wise man who built his house on the rock! And the rain descended, the floods came and the winds blew and beat on that house; and it did not fall for it was founded on the rock".* (Matthew 7:24-27) What Rock? The words of Jesus. He is the rock

Jesus asked His disciples, *"Who do men say I am?" So they answered "some say you are John the Baptist, others say Elijah, others say Jeremiah or one of the prophets" He said to them, "but who do you say that I am?" And Simon Peter answered and said "You are the Christ, the Son of the Living God"* Then Jesus told Peter that his confession was the rock on which Christ's church would be built. (Matthew 16:13-18) Was Peter the rock? No Christ is the Rock. Peter's confession...... the fact that Jesus is the Son of God.....that is the rock on which the church was built.

After Jesus was put to death on the cross, *a rich man from Arimathea named Joseph, who himself had also become a disciple of Jesus, went to Pilate and asked for the body to be given to him. And when Joseph had taken the body, he wrapped it in a clean linen cloth, and laid it in his new tomb which he had hewn out of the rock; and he rolled a large stone against the door of the tomb.* (Matthew 27:57-60) Jesus was buried inside a rock and sealed in with another rock.

But He didn't stay inside that rock! He rose on the third day and even now He is still our Rock!

There is a wonderful lady here at the church who gathers rocks and paints scriptures and pictures on them and gives them away as reminders to the rest of us, of the beautiful story of Christ.

So the next time you are outside, pick up a rock and remember who created it. Remember His Son, your Rock and your Salvation. Then give that rock to someone else and tell them the story.

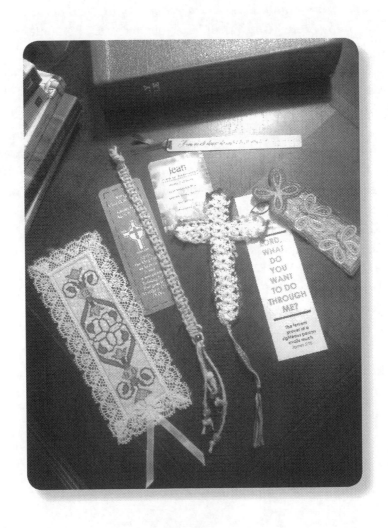

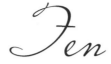

BOOKMARKS

I love books! E-books are OK, but I like the way books feel; the weight of them in my hands. I like the whisper of pages turning, the smell of new editions and the handwritten notes of long ago readers in older volumes.

We didn't always have books. The ancient Egyptians advanced from clay tablets to handwritten scrolls just in time for Moses to record God's history. Later the prophets wrote on scrolls concerning God's laws, and the coming of the Messiah.

In the first century AD, during the time of Herod, the Romans invented the codex. This was an early form of books, more like notebooks. They were hand written pages and drawings sewn together and bound with thin wooden covers. This was just in time for men chosen by God to record the life of Christ and His teachings. Then some of these men and other inspired men wrote letters to the church. Copies were made and carried wherever Christians went, spreading the written word of God into every nation.

Isn't God's timing perfect? But why keep these records? Why write everything down?

King David said his writings were written for generations to come. (Psalms 102:18)

Luke wrote to his friend, Theophilus, *It seems good to me, having had perfect understanding* (a miraculous gift) *of all things from the very first to write to you an orderly account.* (Luke 1:1-3)

The apostle Paul wrote to the church in Rome *For whatever things were written before were written for our learning, that we through the patience and comfort of the Scriptures might have hope.* (Romans 15:4)

The apostle Peter wrote *I now write to you this second epistle (in both of which I stir up your pure minds by way of reminder) that you may be mindful of the words which were spoken before by the holy prophets, and of the commandment of us, the apostles, by the Lord and Savior.* (2 Peter 3:1-2)

God arranged for the history of His creation, all the events that led up to the redemption of mankind and all the instructions needed for Godly living to be preserved on written pages. King David said they were written to teach future generations. Luke said they were written to give us a true account. Paul said they were written to give us hope. Peter said they were written to remind us of all those teachings of the prophets, apostles and Jesus Himself. Now listen to what the apostle John tells us about his writings that God has preserved for us. *These things I have written to you who believe in the name of the Son of God, that you may know that you have eternal life. And that you may continue to believe in the message of the Son of God.* (1John 5:13) How about that for a reason to write something down?! We can know, we don't need to have doubts, we can know..... we have salvation!

Now that we have answered the question of why these things were written down. Now we ask who is the real author?

King David rote, *The eternity of Your word is truth, and every one of Your righteous judgments endures forever. (*Psalms 119:160)

Peter wrote, *Knowing this first, that no prophecy of Scripture is of any private interpretation, for prophecy never came by the will of man, but holy men of God spoke as they were moved by the Holy Spirit.* (2 Peter 1: 20-21)

Paul wrote the same thing to Timothy *All Scripture is given by inspiration of God and is profitable for doctrine, for reproof, for correction, for instruction in righteousness, that the man of God may be complete, thoroughly equipped for every good work.* (2 Timothy 3:16-17)

The writer of the book of Hebrews tells us *For the word of God is living and powerful and sharper than any two edged sword.* (Hebrews 4:12)

King David and the writer of Hebrews said these writings are the words of God. Peter said the men who wrote these words were guided by the Holy Spirit. Paul said all scripture was given by inspiration. There are sixty six book and letters written by God-inspired writers, included in our Bible. All of these books of history and poetry, all of these books of prophecy and teaching, all of these letters of instruction, encouragement and assurance were written by forty men and preserved for us by the Holy Spirit. But there was only one Author, God Himself!

Are all these words worth reading? Are they worth remembering? These inspired words were divinely written and preserved to teach us and remind us of our faith, our hope and our salvation. Are they worth anything to you? Do you cherish them, study them, glean wisdom from them. Are they worth reading? Remembering?

There have been many writers over the years who have sold thousands, even millions of copies of their books, but for almost two thousand years, there have been more copies of God's scripture made available than the writings of any man. How many copies of the Bible are in your house today? How many books of every description? On tables, in shelves, on nightstands, sometimes stacked on the floor or in boxes. At any given time there are half a dozen on the table by "my chair", and all these books have one thing in common....

Book marks! Everyday markers with advertising printed on them. Maybe just a torn scrap of paper with hand written notes, but some of them are works of art; beautiful embroidered fabric, etched brass or crocheted crosses. But the very best have scripture printed on them, maybe the verses we just read.

Evidently Paul was a reader too. Luke records Paul quoting from the Greek poet, Epimenides, *For in Him we live and more and have our being.* And the second part of that verse is a quote from the Cecilian poet, Aratus *For we are also His offspring.* (Acts 17:28) These men were honoring false Gods but Paul took their words to describe the One True God. When Paul wrote to the church in Corinth, he quoted another Greek poet, Menander, *Evil company Corrupts good habits.* (1 Corinthians 15:33) When he wrote to Titus, he again quoted from Epimenides concerning the habits of the Cretans. (Titus 1:12) He said they were all liars. Paul also quoted from many writers of the Old Testament. Eighty four times in the letter to the Roman church alone! So, with all his reading....I wonder how many bookmarks Paul had.

I hope you enjoy reading your Bible as much as I do, and other books as well, and I hope you appreciate all the beautiful bookmarks. Start a project for your children or your Bible class. Have them make Bible book marks, not just for themselves, but make lots of them to give away; to help them remember the greatest of all authors, The Lord God Almighty.

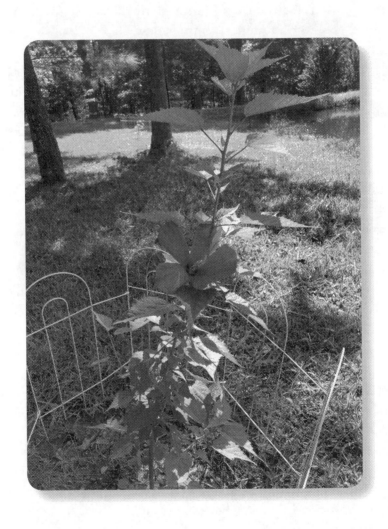

Eleven

FLOWERS AND HERBS

The early years of my growing up were spent in a small town in Ohio with my parents, all my grandparents, some great grandparents, aunts and uncles, great aunts and uncles, and a BUNCH of cousins. One of the things I remember most, is the pride all the women took in their flower gardens.

Mom's mother grew roses. Big, beautiful fragrant roses you could smell from the other side of the yard. Dad's mother had big snow- ball bushes, tiny lily of the valley and hollyhocks we turned into dancing dolls. Her mother had an herb garden and an arbor full of Concord grapes. My mom's aunt had wonderful french lilacs.

In Idaho, Mom had iris of every color all along our driveway and a rose garden just outside the big sliding glass doors in our living room, that always reminded me of my grandmother.

In the Spring, our house in Arkansas is surrounded by the smell of magnolia, a little later it is roses and then gardenia. In the fall the sweet olives begin to bloom and put out their fragrance. When I am working the flower beds and herb garden, I sometimes get lost in time, remembering that small town where my life began.

Herbs and flowers have always been a part of celebrations and used as food, as medicine and as scents. Over time they have developed their own individual symbolic meanings. There is not enough room here to list them all, but some of my favorites are:

Lily of the Valley - In France, it is the harbinger of Spring. Here we think of

Jonquils and Hyacinths.

Lavender is for virtue

Gardenia is the symbol of secret love

Bay leaves, the Romans saw them as a symbol of triumph

Dogwood means everlasting love

Daisy is for innocence and purity

Chrysanthemum symbolize optimism

Alstromeria is the sign of prosperity.

Sage represents a wise man

Daffodils symbolize chivalry

Rosemary is for remembrance

Thyme is for courage

Of course, everyone has their own favorite they associate with a special occasion and or special person.

Flowers and herbs have always been part of the funeral ritual. When Jesus was laid in the tomb, Nicodemus supplied about a hundred pounds of the traditional myrrh, aloes and spices to wrap the body, (John 19:38-40) That following Sunday morning, the women came with additional spices and fragrant oils to further anoint the body. (Luke 23:55-56)

I love to go to weddings! I appreciate all the time and thought that goes into selecting just the right flowers and in some cultures, herbs. It used to be the custom for brides to pick a flower for it's scent and then adopt that scent for her trademark perfume.

When I walk past one of our Rose of Sharon shrubs or the lily bed, I remember a line from the song of Solomon, *"I am the Rose of Sharon and the Lily of the valley"* (Song of Solomon 2:1) This beautiful love story is symbolic of the love Jehovah God had for Israel (Ezekiel 16:8-14) and the love that His Son would have for His church. (Ephesians 5:1-2)

Isaiah was prophesying about the coming of the kingdom (the church) when he said *"the desert shall rejoice and blossom as a rose. It shall blossom abundantly and rejoice. The glory of Lebanon, the best of Carmel and Sharon shall see the glory of the Lord"* (Isaiah 35:1-2)

What were Solomon and Isaiah talking about?

Sharon was a semi desert area just North of Mt. Carmel, not far from the town of Nazareth, where Jesus grew up and it was famous for it's roses. Other valleys around Mt Carmel had fields filled with lilies prized by perfumers. Makers of perfume still use the oil from these flowers to make beautiful scents.

Mt Carmel itself, was considered a place of beauty, park like. Historians believe this is probably the place where Jesus taught His lesson on the Beatitudes. (Matthew 5)

Mt Lebanon grew world renowned cedar trees, some of which were taken to Jerusalem in the days of Solomon to be used in the building of the temple. (1Kings 5:6) The mountain was located just Northwest of Caesarea Philippi where Peter made his confession of faith ***"You are the Christ, the Son of the Living God."*** (Matthew 16:13-17) In the very next chapter, we are told Jesus took Peter, James and John up on a high mountain, believed to be Lebanon, to witness His transfiguration.

Now we understand Solomon using the Rose of Sharon and the Lily of the valley to represent the Lord, and why Isaiah said these these places would see the glory of the Lord. These places did see the glory of the Lord! These places saw the events in the life and death of the Lord and the beginning of the church.

Matthew and Luke both record the lesson Jesus gave about the lilies of the field. Their life is short, He said, but God supplies all they need to grow, bloom and reproduce. Then Jesus asked a question ***"If your Heavenly Father supplies all that lilies need, don't you think He will supply all you need?"*** (Matthew 6:28-31)

The lily has two jobs. One is to produce fragrant flowers, a fragrant aroma. When Noah offered burnt offerings on the altar, the Lord smelled a smoothing aroma. (Genesis 8:21) Later, under the Law of Moses, everyone was expected to bring sacrifices to God. Animal sacrifices, burnt on altars were a pleasing aroma to God, but if the one offering the sacrifice was not a faithful follower of God, ***"I will not smell the fragrance of your sweet aroma"*** (Leviticus 26:31)

Under the new law, the law of Christ, His followers are not instructed to make animal sacrifices to be pleasing to Him. Paul said a man named Epaphroditus brought him a gift from the church in Philippi. ***The things which were sent from you, a sweet smelling aroma, an acceptable sacrifice, well pleasing to God.*** (Philippians 4:18)

Paul told the church in Corinth, ***For we are to God the fragrance of Christ among those who are being saved and among those who are***

perishing. (2 Corinthians 2:15) God wants us to look and "smell" like Christ not only when we are among Christians, but when we are among unbelievers! We, like the lilies, are to produce a sweet smelling aroma which Paul said is our giving gifts to others; our money, our time, our talents, our labor, when we extend love, compassion, mercy and forgiveness. That is our sacrifice, our sweet aroma to God.

The lily's other job is to scatter the seed God gave it, so God can produce more lilies. Have you ever seen lily seed? The lily bed is full of little black seeds when the bloom matures. Some of those seeds fall in our bed, some on the brick wall around the front of the bed, some on the patio on the other side. The lilies are not careful where their seeds fall.

Jesus told a parable about a sower who went out and scattered seed. He scattered it everywhere. All kinds of soil. Some of the seed produced plants and some did not. It wasn't up to the sower. (Mark 4:3-8) Jesus then when on to explain (verses 14-20) that seed is His word and we are the sowers! We are to scatter seeds, EVERYWHERE, so God can produce more Christians. We are to teach others; at home, on the job, at school, in our neighborhoods, at the dentist office, the grocery store. We don't have to preach a sermon to someone to scatter the seed. Just remind them of God and His love for them.

We are to become God's lilies! We are to produce a sweet smelling aroma and scatter seeds. Next time you are in your yard, cut some flowers or herbs, share them with your neighbors and remind them of the one true Rose of Sharon and the perfect Lily of the field.

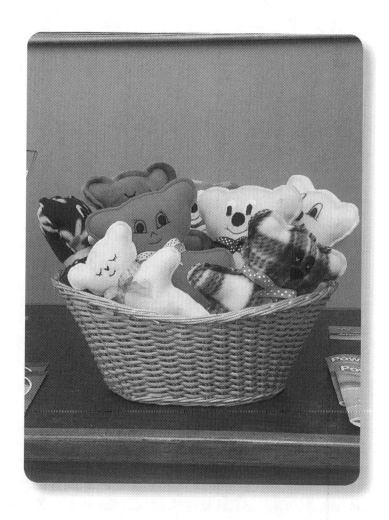

Twelve

RODS AND NEEDLES

"Idle hands are the devil's workshop" I learned this by example; it wasn't just words. My mom and dad learned from their parents and passed it down to us.

"If you can't find something to do, I'll find you something!"

"Whatever you do, do it right the first time."

"When you start a job, always have something else ready to do when you are finished."

My folks taught me well. I never run out of things to do. I am one of those people who, while working on one project, always have several more waiting. Sewing, oil painting, ceramics, baking, all turned into vocations. I like to garden, crochet and cook, and lately I've added writing. I am a detail person. I love a challenge. My paintings show individual leaves on trees and petals on flowers. My crochet projects are intricate, with lots of different stitches and patterns. The more difficult, the better I like it. Some of my friends were studying one of my finished crocheted blankets and I heard one of them say the other, "I wonder what her brain looks like!"

Besides being funny, it made me wonder; what does my brain look like... to my Heaven Father? What does He think of my work? My efforts? The way I use my time? Other people use their brains in different ways; music, sports, other arts and crafts, their jobs become their hobbies or like me, their hobbies become jobs. What does the Bible have to say about the use of our time and our talents? Why do we do all these things? To what purpose? Do we do things just for ourselves? Do we use our time and talents just to please ourselves? What does God want us to do with the talent we have?

Paul said, when you were born into Christ, you were created *for good works which God prepared before time that we should walk in them.* (Ephesians 2:10)

Paul also tells you, not only did God create you to do good works, but He will supply all you need to perform the work you were created to do! *And God is able to make all grace abound toward you, that you, always having all sufficiency in all things, may have an abundance for every good work.* (2 Corinthians 9:8)

But some of you say, "I'm not as good at that as our preacher's wife" or "I don't have talents like other people do". Do you believe Paul was inspired by God? Do you believe what he said? God gave you work to do and everything you need to do it. Now open your Bible. *But let each one examine his own work and then he will have rejoicing in himself alone, and not in another. For each shall bear his own load.* (Galatians 6:4-5) Did you read that? Do not compare yourself to anyone else! Examine your own work. God gave you a work. God will give you what you need, to do the work for which you were created. He expects you to carry your own load. To accomplish you own good works!

The Lord said to Moses, *"What is that you have in your hand?" And Moses replied a rod"* A common tool that every shepherd had. God said "Use it for Me I will help you." (Exodus 4:1-5) And He did! That rod helped Moses lead the children of Israel out of Egypt and through the wilderness. (Exodus 7:8-13; 14:13-31; 17:5-6)

Dorcas used the needle that was in her hand to serve God. She made clothing for the poor and the widows. (Acts 9:36)

The Hebrew writer tells us, God remembers our good works. (Hebrews 6:10) It isn't enough to say we love God or Jesus, we have to SHOW it. It isn't enough to say you love anyone, you have to SHOW it. *My little children, let us not love in word or tongue, but in deeds and in truth.* (1John 3:18)

It isn't enough to say we believe in the existence of God. It isn't enough to say we believe what He said or what Jesus said. It isn't enough to say we believe the instructions given by the inspired apostles. We have to live our lives SHOWING our faith. Not only do we show our love by our deeds, but we show our faith the same way. *So also, faith by itself, if it does not have good works, is dead.* (James 2:14-18). James did not say your good works would save you! But he did say faith by itself is no good. We show our love and our faith by our good deeds.

Hebrews, chapter eleven is the "faith passage" in your Bible. In the first thirty two verses we find listed our heroes of faith. Nineteen men and women are named along with the stories of how their faith provided love, obedience and good works. The rest of the chapter is a list of trials people had endured because of their faith and we can read all of these stories of faith in the pages of our Bible.

God has always required love, faith and good works toward Him and for our families, friends, neighbors, church family and those around us.

God has always used His people to teach, to set the example and to serve others, just as Abraham, Moses and the prophets did, just as Jesus, the apostles and early Christians did.

Isaiah told the Israelites. *"Learn to do good"* (Isaiah 1:17)

Jesus said *"Let your light so shine before men, that they may see your good works and glorify your Father in Heaven.* (Matthew 5:16)

Matthew tells us about the occasion when Mary anointed Jesus and He said *"She has done a good work for Me"* (Matthew 26:6-13)

Paul wrote to the church in Colosse, gain wisdom and understanding *that you may have a walk worthy of the Lord, fully pleasing Him, being fruitful in every good work and increasing in the knowledge of God.* (Colossians 1:10)

Paul instructed the young preacher, Timothy, to tell the wealthy in his congregation *to do good, not to be haughty, nor to trust in uncertain riches but in the living God, who gives us richly all things to enjoy. Let them do good that they may be rich in good works, ready to give, ready to share storing up for themselves a good foundation for the time to come, that they may lay hold on eternal life.* (1Timothy 6:17-19) He wasn't talking about just millionaires. By their standard, all of us are rich! A lot of the Christians of the first century were slaves or misplaced people and it was up to those who had the means to help, to help them. And we don't have to be millionaires to help others. We just need to share whatever we have.

Luke tells us *Jesus went about doing good.* (Acts 10:38) Do you have a better example to follow as a pattern for your life?

What does your brain look like to your Father? What does He see you thinking about? Are you thinking of others and how you can serve them? Are you working, preparing to serve them?

What's in your hand? A needle? A sewing machine? A soup pot? A garden rake? Maybe you are an encourager, like Barnabas; (Acts 4:36) maybe a Bible teacher, like Priscilla and her husband; (Acts 18) or a hostess, like Mary. (John 12:1-2) There are places you can volunteer; homeless establishments, schools, hospitals for a start. There are ministries in your congregation that could use help. If not, start one. One of the ministries of the church here is the "Bear ministry" several ladies make little bears for the local hospitals and a children's advocacy center. They also send them to Africa and Mexico and give them away at their church building.

Through good works and kindness you will show your love and your faith to your family, your co-workers, your church family and even total strangers. You may be the only example of Godly love that person will see today. There are those around you who are walking through this world with heavy burdens and struggles you don't know about. This could be the day they really need an encouraging word, a smile or a helping hand. Take time as you walk through your day, to notice. Is your cashier at the grocery store, or your waitress at the cafe looking stressed? Does your doctor or the kid's teacher look like they are at the end of their rope sometimes? Don't pry, just tell them how much you appreciate their work. Give them a smile. Take your druggist a box of donuts just because he was so helpful, when you were stressed! How about the man who helped you with your computer when it just would not co-operate? Did you just take it for granted that was his job, or did you really thank him for saving your work and your pictures for you?! He deserved a box of donuts too! Maybe these folks need to be reminded of the love that comes from good people and the love and provision that their Heavenly Father offers.

Don't say you can't. Try. Use what God gave you, whatever it is....and get busy! You be the reminder God needs. He will help you.

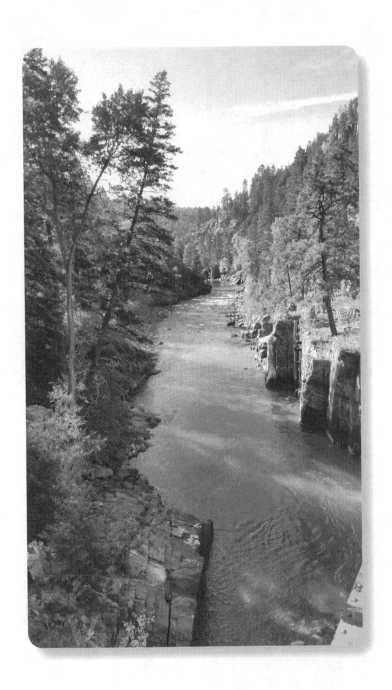

Thirteen

WATER

To sit by the ocean early in the morning and watch the sun rise as it comes closer and closer, growing larger and larger, and brighter and brighter until it bursts clear of the water and reflects off the crashing waves, that is awe-inspiring.

To drink from an icy cold mountain river where the water is so deep and yet so clear you can see the bottom, that is amazing.

To listen to the babbling of a spring as it makes it's was through the forest, that is tranquility.

To watch a waterfall is to see beauty.

When she was little, my granddaughter, Kenzie, would come to see me and ask "can we prinkle today?" Translation: "Can we turn on the lawn sprinkler and watch the robins play?" And the two of us would sit and laugh as we watched the robins play in the sun-sparkled water. That sprinkler brought us hours of pleasure and God supplied all the water we needed from our well.

Water. It speaks to us. It tells us of God's love, power, provision and His salvation. There are more than seven hundred references to water found in the Bible. We are going to explore some of those passages and find messages from God.

In the very beginning God's Spirit moved over the waters to prepare a home for mankind. And the Spirit of God was hovering over the face of the waters And then God said **"Let the waters under the heavens be gathered together into one place and let the dry land appear." and it was so.** (Genesis 1:1-10)

Moses told us about God using water to save the children of Israel from their enemy. They had decided to follow Moses out of four hundred years of bondage in Egypt and go back home to Canaan. They were on their way when they looked ahead and saw the Red Sea in front of them and behind them, the Egyptian army was following. When all seemed lost, God rolled back the waters of the Red Sea and the Israelites walked through the sea on dry land. Then God turned the water loose and it came thundering back to destroy Pharaoh's army, but God's people were safe on the other side. (Exodus 14:21-23)

God used water to show His power through physical healing. Naaman was a powerful, influential man, he was a commander in the Syrian army but he was also a leper. (2 Kings 5) When he was told about a prophet in Samaria who could heal him, he went to see the prophet. And he went prepared to pay enough silver and gold to equal over three million dollars of our money today to get what he wanted. He was expecting a great ceremony and an awe inspiring miraculous production to heal him and he was quite willing to pay for it. When Naaman arrived at Elisha's house, a servant gave him a message from Elisha with instructions to go wash in the Jordan river seven times in order to be healed. That was it. No charge, no big production.... just go wash. Naaman was furious! "Who does this prophet think he is!? Having a servant tell me what to do! Telling me to go get in that filthy river! I expect him to come himself and give me respect and honor and have a show of my healing." He was so angry, he left!

Naaman's servant convinced him to do as he was told and when he did go into the Jordan river as instructed, he was completely healed! No big production, no show, no money needed. Just do what God said and have faith that He will do what He said He would do.

The apostle John tells us about a blind man who received his sight when he followed the instructions of Jesus and washed in the pool of Siloam. (John 9:6-7)

Before he was a king, the boy David was a shepherd and he knew sheep would not drink from running water because of the danger of being swept away. After he became King of Israel, David said his Lord was a good shepherd because He led him to the safety of still waters. (Psalm 23:2) David didn't need a safe place to bathe or get a drink, he needed the inner safety and peace found in his Lord.

The Lord told His people *"If you had heeded my commandment! Then your peace would have been like a river."* (Isaiah 48:18)

The Lord directed His people to *"let their justice run down like water And righteousness like a mighty stream."* (Amos 5:24)

God told Jeremiah *"My people have forsaken Me, the Fountain of Living Waters" (Jeremiah 2:13)* This is the same Living Water Jesus offered! He told the woman at Jacob's well, *"who ever drinks of the water that I shall give him will never thirst. But the water I shall give him will become in him a fountain of water springing up into everlasting life."* (John 4:14) What is this water Jesus offered? The words of God. His teachings.

We've studied the account of Noah and the ark and the power of the Almighty God who used water to destroy a sin filled world. But He used that same water to raise the ark and Noah above the destruction! (Genesis chapters 6, 7 and 8) When the apostle Peter described the circumstances of the flood and the ark, he said, this is the same way baptism destroys your sins and saves you! *"There is also an antitype* (of Noah) *which now saves us, namely baptism (not the removal of the filth of the flesh but the answer of a good conscience toward God")* (1Peter 3:20-21)

Baptism destroys all the sins of your past while at the same time raising you up new and clean. The water doesn't wash the dirt from your body but, because of your faith.... that God will do what He says He will.....He washes and saves your soul and your sins are destroyed in the waters of baptism. The same way Noah was saved and the wicked destroyed by the same water. The same way the Israelites were saved but their enemy was destroyed by the same water.

God uses water for His purposes, but, IT IS ALWAYS HIS POWER THAT ACCOMPLISHES THE DEED! He uses water to remind us of His power, His guidance, His justice, peace, healing, provision, destruction and salvation.

But your salvation is not the end of the story.

Open your Bible to John 7:37-38 *"If anyone thirsts, let him come to Me and drink. And if he believes in Me, as the scripture has said, out of his heart will flow rivers of living water."* Read that again. Now read verse 39. *But this He spoke concerning the Spirit whom those believing in Him would receive; for the Holy Spirit was not yet given, because Jesus was not yet glorified.*

Jesus said there would come a time, after His death, resurrection and ascension back to heaven (that is when He would be glorified) that His believers would be the source of living water! And we read about it happening for the first time in Acts 2:38 Then Peter said to them *"repent and let every one of you be baptized in the name of Jesus Christ for the remission of sins; and you shall receive the gift of the Holy Spirit."* At their baptism, the Holy Spirit, the Living Water was given to each of them. And what was that living water? Salvation through the words of Jesus. His message of saving grace.

And it still happens today. When you believe in Christ as the Son of God and are baptized into Him and become a Christian; when you receive the gift of the Holy Spirit, out of your heart will flow the living water. You become the source of the living water! If you let Him, God will use you to spread the words of Jesus, His words of salvation, His truth. You become the reminder to those around you.

Remind them of the One True God and His power of salvation.

A LAST FEW WORDS

We need to remember what we have received from our Heavenly Father, the beauty of His creation and the very breath of life within us, His love and protection, His care and provision, His forgiveness and His salvation, His everlasting words. In his letter to the Romans (Romans 5:21-21), Paul reminds his readers that because of Christ and His death, we were given these things. We don't deserve these things and we cannot buy or earn any of these things. They are all wrapped up in one word GRACE, which we receive through our Lord, Jesus Christ and it was freely given to all people. (verse18)

But most people do not accept the gift because along with the gift comes a life of responsibility. A life that is patterned after the Giver. And He said *"If you love Me, keep my commandment"* (John 14:15) If we love Him we will do all we can to keep all of His commands. Not just the ones that are convenient, not just the ones we are in the mood to follow, not just the ones we feel are right, but all of them, all of the time, to the best of our ability.

One of the commands He gave was to love each other. *A new commandment I give you, that you love one another as I have loved you, that you also love one another.* (John 13:34) How many examples did He give us, of showing love to others? How many examples did He give of going about doing good? The recorded life of Jesus tells what this love looks like. He showed what forgiveness, compassion, mercy, service and obedience look like. And He told us to show love in the same way.

So as you walk through this life, you are to remember all that Jesus said and did, so you can do the same. That is a tall order and you will not do it perfectly every time. But, does that mean you are not to try at all? It will not be easy. But, it will be impossible if you don't spend time with Him and learn all you can about Him. Spend time in His Word, and then remember what you have read and put it into practice.

But, it isn't enough for you to remember. Who will remind your children? Your grandchildren? Your neighbors, friends and family? Will the preacher? the Bible class teacher? or your mother? Don't depend on someone else to remind them. God told you, it was your responsibility. You remind them.

The Lord bless you and keep you: The Lord make His face to shine upon you, And be gracious to you; The Lord lift up His countenance upon you and give you peace. (Numbers 6:24-26)

May God bless you in your walk with Him.

Jean Melson

BIOGRAPHY

Jean taught her first Bible class at age sixteen and has never stopped. She majored in English at Idaho State University and Magic Valley Christian College. Since then she has worn many hats; teacher, artist, wife, mother, florist, co-owner of "I Do" Weddings, grandmother, gardener, bride for the second time and great grandmother.

She has taught in Bible classes and Bible camps across the U.S., in Africa, Mexico and Ukraine.

She and her husband, Mike live on three and a half acres in the beautiful Hot Springs, Arkansas area and spend time working outside and enjoying the beauty God gave them.

They work and worship with the Village Church of Christ and are living a blessed life.

Printed in the United States
By Bookmasters